Ketogenic Diet:

Conquering Diabetes with Ketogenic Diet

Table of Contents

Introduction

This book contains proven steps and strategies on how to conquer diabetes with ketogenic diet. Ketogenic diet is the ideal diet for you to lose weight naturally, remain disease free and improve your overall health. Countless dieters around the world are following this low carb, high fat diet to improve their health and lose weight.

Ketogenic diet is based on foods that are low in carb and high in fat and protein. Beside weight loss this diet will help you to lower heart disease, stabilize cholesterol, prevent stroke and various cancers. As a diabetic patient, the ketogenic diet is perfect for you because it is incredibly effective reversing diabetes.

These days most people are following a typical diet plan that consists high amount of carb and sugar rich foods. This is the reason why so many people are suffering from chronic inflammation and developed insulin resistance. Sadly, their bodies have lost the ability to burn excess fat and carbohydrates consumed through diet are lowering their liver function.

Ketogenic diet will assist you to reverse diabetes and help your body to become insulin sensitive again. Following the diet will train your body to become an efficient fat burning machine within a couple of weeks.

Chapter 1 What is Ketogenic Diet

Starting the ketogenic diet is one of the easiest ways for you to conquer type II diabetes and avoid other diseases. The ketogenic diet was introduced in 1920's to stop pediatric epilepsy in children. Doctors thought that ketogenic diet prevents seizures. The ketogenic diet became hugely popular among general population when researchers demonstrated in 1990's that the diet is beneficial for adults also.

 The ketogenic diet offers you diet that is low in carbohydrate, moderate protein and high in fat. The diet will effectively train your body to burn fat instead of carbohydrate to produce energy. With fat based diet, your body will have more fuel to burn during the day and help you remain active throughout the day.

The diet will help you to shred body fat and lose steady weight naturally. To understand how ketogenic or keto diet works, you have to know how ketosis works. Ketosis is the foundation of the ketogenic diet. The fat you take via ketogenic diet is transformed into fatty acids, then processed by the liver and send back to the blood as ketones; your body then uses ketones as glucose sugar instead of glucose generated by carbohydrate rich foods.

When your body is in a ketosis state, meaning that your body is breaking down body fat to produce the energy it needs. It also means that your body is converting fat to generate energy instead of carbohydrate.

Types of ketogenic diet

There are basically 4 types of ketogenic diets:

- o Standard Ketogenic Diet or SKD: SKD is a basic ketogenic diet, in this diet you eat the minimum amount of carbohydrate continually. If you are not maintaining an active life, then consume 20 to 50 grams of carbs to follow this diet.

- o Targeted Ketogenic Diet or TKD: TKD is an old approach to follow the ketogenic diet. With this diet plan you eat carb rich foods 30 to 60 minutes before exercise and carbs are effectively burned during the exercise. After exercise, you can eat foods that are high in protein and low in fat.

- o New Approach or TKD: Various recent studies have revealed that consuming carbs just before exercise may not be helpful. Dr Volek and Dr Phinney in their book "The Art and Science of Low Carbohydrate Performance" mentions that you don't have to consume extra carbs before exercise.

- Cyclic Ketogenic Diet or CKD: CKD is mainly for bodybuilders and athletes. In this diet plan athletes and bodybuilders consume carbohydrate rich foods one day (450 to 600 grams) and consume a ketogenic diet subsequent day to maximize fat-loss and building less muscle mass.

Ketogenic diet and health benefits

Ketogenic diet helps you to lose weight and lowers your risk of various other health conditions. There is scientific evidence that ketogenic diet helps with:

- Obesity

- Type II Diabetes

- Epilepsy

Research is still continuing, but it is strongly believed that ketogenic diet helps with acne, polycystic ovaries, neurological diseases and some cancers. Athletes recommend that following ketogenic diet enhances endurance.

Ketogenic diet and reversing type II diabetes

Ideally you want to remain healthy and prevent any type of health problem in life. You have to methodically regulate your blood sugar and insulin levels to reverse one of the major disease of modern times, type II diabetes. These days, diabetes is becoming a major health problem for both youngsters and adults.

When you consume a typical carbohydrate rich meal, with the exception of fiber, your body breaks all other elements to glucose. Glucose mixes in the blood and triggers the release of insulin in the body. Habitually eating foods that are high in carbohydrate and refined sugar, spikes glucose and insulin levels in the body. This condition escalates the risk of developing insulin resistance in the body and eventually leads to type II diabetes.

The magic of ketogenic diet

Unlike carbohydrate and refined sugars, fat doesn't trigger a spike in glucose or insulin levels in your body. The diet trains your body to burn fat to produce energy instead of glucose. So surplus glucose or insulin release in your body is avoided and your diabetic is reversed!

Tips for the beginners

1. One of the main goals of the ketogenic diet to limit carbohydrate intake. Your goal should be to eat less than 20g daily. With the help of the internet, you can easily measure your carb intake and don't have to worry about eating too much carb rich foods.

2. A ketogenic diet contains 60 to 75% fat, 15 to 30% protein and 5 to 10%

carbohydrates. The internet is a great help for you to calculate and measure your meals.

3. With ketogenic or keto diet you are eating less carb, but careful about eating too much protein. Surplus protein can cause higher levels of insulin production.

4. You have to strictly follow the ketogenic diet and can't break the routine even for a day. If you break the routine, then you have to again start from the beginning.

5. If you are not certain about any food or food item, check and check again before consuming it.

6. Avoid root vegetables because they are loaded with carb.

7. For the beginner's it is sensible to drink a cup of broth daily for the first couple of weeks. Consuming broth will help you to maintain electrolyte balance in your body and avoid keto flu.

8. Before you start the diet, take some picture of yourself from all angles and compare them after 1 month. The difference in body shape will encourage you to keep going with the keto diet for life.

9. Read articles about the keto diet in the newspaper and on the internet. Also

read e-books, watch videos to know as much as possible about the diet.

Tips for maintaining a ketogenic diet for life

Often people can't stick to a certain diet because it demands them to avoid eating foods that they enjoy. However, if you follow a ketogenic diet, you only have to eliminate carbohydrate rich foods. This is the reason the ketogenic diet is easy to maintain. Following are some useful tips for you to maintain the diet for life:

o Find someone who can give you mental support when starting the diet. The person might be your friend or a family member. Someone who continues to encourage you will help you to stay focused on the diet.

o Consult with your doctor if you feel you need supplements and added vitamins.

o Mix things up and try a variety of recipes every week. This way you will have different foods to taste every day. Diet will be exciting and unpredictable and you will find it easier to follow.

o Experiment with the ingredients. Experiment and create your own ketogenic recipes, use food items that you enjoy to eat. Experimenting will keep you interested in the diet.

o Drink lots of water, this will help remove toxins and other waste materials from your body. Water will also make you feel full and help you control craving for foods that are not included in the diet.

o Follow a fixed timetable for sleep and ensure that you are getting a satisfactory amount of sleep daily. Studies have revealed that people eat more when they are tired or sleep deprived. When you are regularly sleeping for a short period of time, your body starts to produce a hormone name ghrelin that force you to overeat.

o Eat 5-6 smaller meals daily and ensure that you are not too hungry anytime. If you are starving, naturally you will go for sugar and carb rich foods and lose the benefits of the ketogenic diet.

Chapter 2 Foods That Are Allowed and Prohibited in Ketogenic Diet

The goal of the ketogenic diet is to train your body to produce energy from fat rich foods instead of carbohydrate and sugar rich foods. The quality of the food is also important, especially when it comes to protein and fat rich foods. Buy meats that are organic, grass-fed and pasture-raised, choose butter creams, and cheese from grass-fed source, buy organically produce vegetables, fruits and eggs.

1. Fats and Oils: Fats and oils are the base of the ketogenic diet and you have to eat a plenty of fats and oils. As you know certain fats and oils are better for you than others. Consume a high amount of saturated fats in the form of meat, poultry, eggs, butter and coconut oil; monounsaturated fats such as nuts and nut butter, olive oil and avocado; natural polyunsaturated fats, such as tuna, and salmon. Avoid highly process polyunsaturated fats such as vegetable oil, canola oil and soybean oil. You can add homemade mayonnaise to your foods as a healthy fat.

2. Proteins: You have to careful when consuming protein because body converts excess amounts of protein into

glucose. Eat bacon, sausage, meat, poultry, eggs, fish, nuts and butter for protein.

3. Dairy: Consume full-fat dairy products such as heavy cream, sour cream, butter, cream cheese, hard cheese, and cottage cheese. Avoid low-fat dairy products and flavored dairy products, such as fruity and flavored yogurt.

4. Vegetables and Fruits: When consuming fruits, you have to limit your intake because most of them are full of natural sugars and regularly consuming them will trigger spikes in blood glucose levels. Choose fruits such as berries. Vegetables are an important element of ketogenic diet because they provide vitamins and essential minerals and most of them don't contain a lot of calories. Focus on vegetables that are low in carbohydrates. Choose mostly dark green and leafy green vegetables such as cucumbers, spinach, broccoli, asparagus, lettuce and green beans. Cauliflower and mushrooms are good for ketogenic diet. Avoid starchy vegetables such as corn, white potatoes, sweet potatoes and yams.

5. Grains and Sugars: Completely avoid all forms of grains and sugars, including wheat, rye, sorghum, barley, rice and any products made from these grains. This basically means no rice, no bread,

no crackers and no pasta. Avoid consuming sugar and anything that contains sugar, such as white and brown sugar, corn, brown rice and maple syrup and honey. Careful when buying packaged foods because a lot of food items contain sugar.

6. Soft Drinks: Drink unsweetened coffee or tea or with an approved sweetener such as Erythritol or stevia. Avoid flavored water, lemonade, fruit juices and sodas.

7. Water: When following the ketogenic diet, drinking sufficient amount of water is extremely important. Ketogenic diet results in more ketones and sodium excreted through your urine than normal. Drink minimum 8 glasses of water daily and add salt to your dishes to maintain a healthy level of electrolytes. Here are a few tips for you to keep your body hydrated:

   ▪ Eat foods that are high in water like celery and cucumber

   ▪ Drink a glass of water in the morning and before bed

   ▪ Carry a bottle of water with you

8. Alcohol: Drink alcohol in moderation because ketogenic diet lowers your alcohol tolerance. Also careful about

carbohydrate and extra calories. Drink a glass of water when consuming alcohol.

9. Spices: Spices are low in carbohydrates and rich in flavor. Dry spices and fresh herbs are encouraged in the ketogenic diet. However, you have to be careful when using prepackaged rubs, flavorings and dried marinades because many prepackaged spice mixes contain sugar and carbohydrate thickening bonding agents and you should avoid them.

10. Sauces: Most of the sauces available in the market contain sugar, so check the label before buying any sauces. For example, tomato sauce can contain as much as 1g of sugar per serving. Following is a list of keto-friendly sauces.

- Cheese sauce

- Béarnaise

- Buffalo sauce

- Alfredo sauce, thickener-free

- Barbecue sauce, sugar-free

- Pasta sauce, sugar-free

- Pizza sauce, sugar-free

- Chimichurri

- Curry

- Pesto

- Cream sauce

- Hollandaise sauce

- Horseradish sauce

11. Condiments: Just like sauces, condiments too generally contain sugar. Many ketchups, salad dressings and marinades are full with sugar. Here are some keto-friendly condiments for you:

   - Capers

   - Ketchup, sugar free

   - Worcestershire sauce, sugar-free

   - Soy sauce

   - Mayonnaise

   - Hot sauce

   - Dill pickle relish

   - Garlic chili paste

   - Salsa, most varieties

   - Mustard, unsweetened

   - Vinegar, cider or most clear varieties

Web help to increase your interest on the ketogenic diet

When following the keto diet, you have to keep track of what you are eating. Without an accurate record, ketogenic diet won't work for you. Some online tools for you to help you with your diet:

- o   Lose It!

- o   Fatsecret

- o   CRON-O-Meter

- o   MyFitnessPal

Following websites will help you to get information about food's nutritional content:

- o   CalorieCount

- o   Fooducate

- o   SELFNutrionData

- o   CalorieKing

Following companies and distributors will help you get low-carb tortillas, low-carb baking mixes, and keto-friendly sauces:

- o   Linda's Diet Delites

- Great Low Carb Bread Company
- Netrition
- Low Carb Connoisseur
- Vitacost

Chapter 3 Breakfast Recipes

Avocado Breakfast Tacos

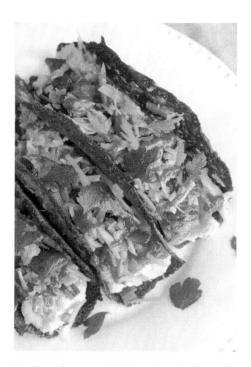

Each photo of this book is taken from ruled.me

Ingredients for 3 servings

- o 6 large Eggs

- 1/2 small Avocado

- 1 oz. Cheddar Cheese, shredded

- 3 strips Bacon

- 2 tbsp. Butter

- 1 cup Mozzarella Cheese, shredded

- Salt and Pepper to Taste

Method

1. Line a baking sheet with foil, put the bacon strips on the baking sheet and bake in the oven at 375F for 15-20 minutes.

2. While the bacon is baking; on a clean pan, heat 1/3 cup of mozzarella at a time, the cheese will act as taco shells.

3. Heat for 2-3 minutes or until the cheese is browned on the edges.

4. With a spatula, unstick the cheese from the pan and then use a pair of tongs to lift the shell up and place it over a wooden spoon resting on a bowl. Repeat with the rest of the cheese.

5. Cook the eggs with butter, stir occasionally. Season with salt and pepper.

6. Spoon 1/3 of the scramble eggs into each cheese shell.

7. Top with sliced avocado and then chopped bacon strips.

8. Sprinkle cheddar cheese over the top of the tacos. Add hot sauce and cilantro if you want.

9. Enjoy.

Nutrition per serving

- o Calorie 443
- o Carbs 3g
- o Fat 36.2g
- o Protein 25.7g

Pumpkin Muffins

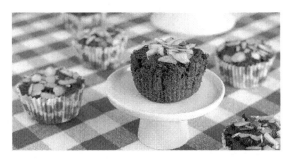

Ingredients for 6 muffins

- o 1 large Egg

- o 1 cup Golden Flaxseed Meal

- o 1 tbsp. Cinnamon

- o 1/2 cup Pumpkin Puree

- o 1/4 cup Slivered Almonds

- o 1 tsp. Vanilla Extract

- o 1/4 cup Sugar-free Caramel Syrup

- o 1 tsp. Apple Cider Vinegar

- o 1/4 cup Cocoa Powder

- o 1/2 tbsp. Baking Powder

- o 1/2 tsp. Salt

- o 2 tbsp. Coconut Oil

Method

1. Preheat the oven to 350F.

2. Combine all the dry ingredients in a deep mixing bowl and mix well.

3. Combine all the wet ingredients in another bowl.

4. Pour the wet ingredients into the dry and mix well to combine.

5. Line a muffin tin with paper liners and spoon ¼ cup of batter into each muffin liner. Sprinkle slivered almonds over the top of each muffin, and lightly press so they are set.

6. Bake in the oven for 15 minutes, or until you see the muffins rise and set on top.

7. Enjoy.

Nutrition per serving

- o Calorie 183
- o Carbs 3.3g
- o Fat 13.4g
- o Protein 7g

Jalapeno Egg Cups

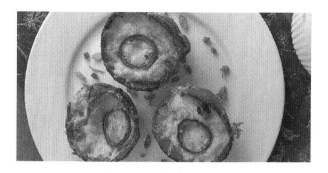

Ingredients for 12 egg cups

- o 8 large Eggs
- o 3 medium Jalapeno Peppers, and 1 for garnish (de-seeded and chopped)
- o 4 oz. Cheddar Cheese
- o 12 strips Bacon
- o 1/2 tsp. Onion Powder
- o 1/2 tsp. Garlic Powder
- o 3 oz. Cream Cheese
- o Salt and Pepper to Taste

Method

1. Preheat the oven to 375F.

2. Pre-cook bacon in a pan so it's semi crisp but still pliable. Keep the bacon grease in the pan.

3. With a hand mixer, mix together chopped and de-seeded jalapeno peppers, eggs, leftover bacon grease, cream cheese, garlic powder, onion powder, and salt and pepper to taste.

4. Grease wells of a muffin tin. Put the pre-cooked bacon around the edges of the wells.

5. Pour egg mixture into the wells of the muffin tin. When baked, the muffins will rise quite a lot, so fill the wells about half-way.

6. Add cheddar and jalapeno slices on top. Bake at 375F for 20-25 minutes.

7. Remove from the oven and set aside to cool.

8. Enjoy.

Nutrition per serving

o Calorie 216
o Carbs .9g
o Fat 19.3g
o Protein 9.6g

Chapter 4 Lunch Recipes

Pepperoni Pizza

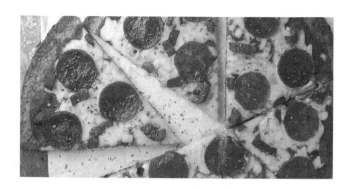

Ingredients for 6 slices of Pepperoni Pizza

Pizza Base

- o   3 tbsp. Cream Cheese (1.5 oz.)
- o   1 tbsp. Psyllium Husk Powder
- o   2 cups Mozzarella Cheese (8 oz.)
- o   1 large Egg
- o   3/4 cup Almond Flour
- o   1 tbsp. Italian Seasoning
- o   1/2 tsp. Salt
- o   1/2 tsp. Pepper

Toppings

- o 1 cup Mozzarella Cheese (4 oz.)
- o 1/2 cup Rao's Tomato Sauce
- o 16 slices Pepperoni
- o Sprinkled Oregano (optional)

Method

1. Melt mozzarella in the microwave
2. In a bowl, mix all base ingredients, except olive oil.
3. Knead the pizza dough into a ball
4. Spread out the pizza dough into a circle using the olive oil on the outside of the dough.
5. Bake the crust under 400F for 10 minutes.
6. Remove the crust from the oven, flip it and bake for another 3-4 minutes.
7. Top the crust with toppings, then bake for additional 4-5 minutes.
8. Allow to cool slightly, slice and serve.

Nutrition per serving

- Calorie 335
- Carbs 3.2g
- Fat 27g
- Protein 18.2g

Almond Flour Mozzarella Egg Sandwich

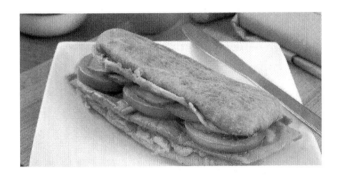

Ingredients for 4 servings

Bread

- o   3/4 cup Almond Flour
- o   2 cups Mozzarella Cheese
- o   1 large Egg
- o   1 tbsp. Psyllium Husk Powder
- o   3 tbsp. Cream Cheese
- o   1/2 tsp. Pepper
- o   1/2 tsp. Salt

Omelette

- o   2 1/2 tbsp. Unsalted Butter

- o 4 tbsp. Ground Beef

- o 2 large Eggs

- o 1/2 small Onion, diced

- o 1 tbsp. Coconut Oil

- o 1 clove Garlic, finely chopped

- o 1 tsp. Water

- o 2 tbsp. chopped Green Onion

- o 1/4 tsp. Curry Powder

- o 2 tbsp. chopped Cilantro

- o 2 tbsp. Mayonnaise (optional)

- o 2 tbsp. Reduced Sugar Ketchup (optional)

- o 3 slices Tomatoes (garnish)

- o 1-piece Butter Lettuce (garnish)

- o 5 slices Cucumber (garnish)

- o Salt and Pepper to Taste

Method

1. Preheat the oven to 400F.

2. Follow the steps of the previous Pepperoni Pizza, excluding the Italian seasoning. Split the dough and shape

into 2 long buns, bake for 30-40 minutes.

3. While the dough is in the oven, prepare the beef. Melt coconut oil in a pan and sauté diced onions until soft and translucent, then add chopped garlic and sauté until fragrant.

4. Add curry powder, water and cook the curry powder for 2 minutes. Add ground beef and season with salt and pepper.

5. Remove the buns from the oven. When they are cooled, slice them horizontally, but don't separate them completely. Spread ½ tbsp. butter onto each bun. Toast the buttered side on a pan.

6. Mix an egg, 1 tbsp. cilantro and 1 tbsp. green onion with half of the cooked beef. Season with salt and pepper. Mix well.

7. Melt 1 tbsp. butter in a pan and add the omelette mixture. Cover the omelette with a bun instantly. Flip and toast the bun when the omelette is cooked.

8. Spread the sauce onto the omelette, garnish with cucumber, tomatoes and lettuce.

9. Repeat the process with other buns and serve.

Nutrition per serving

- o Calorie 620
- o Carbs 6.8g
- o Fat 53.3g
- o Protein 26g

Chicken-Cream Sandwich

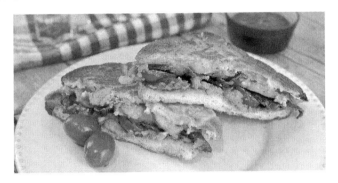

Ingredients for 2 servings

Bread

- o 1/8 tsp. Cream of Tartar
- o 3 oz. Cream Cheese
- o 3 large Eggs
- o 1/4 tsp. Salt
- o 1/2 tsp. Garlic Powder

Filling

- o 2 slices Pepper Jack Cheese
- o 2 Grape Tomatoes
- o 1/4 medium Avocado (about 2 oz.)
- o 2 slices Bacon
- o 1 tsp. Sriracha

- o   1 tbsp. Mayonnaise

- o   3 oz. Chicken

Method

1. Preheat the oven to 300F

2. Separate eggs into 3 different bowls.

3. Add cream of tartar and salt to the whites and whip until foamy peaks form.

4. In another bowl, beat yolks and cream cheese until a pale yellow color.

5. Gently fold the egg whites into the cheese-yolk mixture, half at a time.

6. Scoop ¼ cup batter on a baking sheet lined with parchment paper. Form into square shape and sprinkle garlic over the top of the batter.

7. Bake for 25 minutes.

8. Cook the chicken and the bacon, season with salt and pepper.

9. Assemble the sandwich with mayo, halved tomatoes, sriracha, cheese and mashed avocado.

Nutrition per serving

- o Calorie 361
- o Carbs 2g
- o Fat 28.3g
- o Protein 22g

Chapter 5 Dinner Recipes

Buffalo Chicken Soup

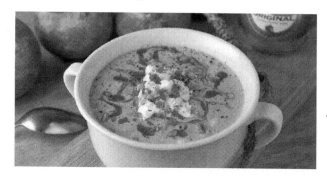

Ingredients for 5 servings

- o   2 oz. Cream Cheese

- o   1/3 – 1/2 cup Hot Sauce

- o   3 medium Chicken Thighs, deboned and sliced (1.2 lbs without bones)

- o   3 cups Beef Broth

- o   1/4 cup Butter

- o   1 cup Heavy Cream

- o   1 tsp. Garlic Powder

- o   1 tsp. Onion Powder

- o   1/4 tsp. Xanthan Gum

- o   1/2 tsp. Celery Seed
- o   Salt and Pepper to Taste

Method

1. De-bone the chicken thighs, then slice them into chunks. Except the xanthan gum, cream and cheese, place the rest of the ingredients in a crockpot with the chicken thighs.

2. Set crockpot on how heat for 6 hours or high heat for 3 hours and let it cook completely.

3. When cooked, remove the chicken and shred with a fork.

4. Add cheese, cream and xanthan gum to the crockpot and emulsify all the liquids together with an immersion blender.

5. Put the chicken back into the crockpot, stir to mix.

6. Season with hot sauce and extra salt and pepper if you want.

Nutrition per serving

- Calorie 523
- Carbs 3.4g
- Fat 44.5g
- Protein 20.8g

Cheddar Cheese Inside Out Burger

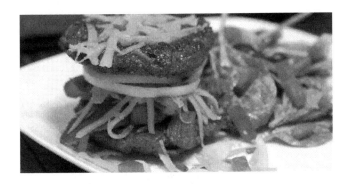

Ingredients for 6 servings of 1 ½ Burgers

- 800g (28 Oz) Ground Beef
- 1/4 Cup Cheddar Cheese
- 2 Tbsp. Chopped Chives
- 8 Slices Chopped Bacon
- 1 Tbsp. Soy Sauce
- 1 tsp. Worcestershire
- 2 tsp. Black Pepper
- 1 tsp. Onion Powder
- 2 tsp. Minced Garlic
- 1 1/4 tsp. Salt

Method

1. In a cast iron skillet, cook the chopped bacon until crisp. Remove when cooked and place on paper towel. Drain the bacon grease separately and save.

2. In a large mixing bowl, combine ground beef,2/3 chopped bacon and rest of the spices.

3. Mix the meat and spices well, divide the mixture and form 9 patties.

4. In the skillet, place 2 tbsp. bacon fat. Put 3-4 patties at a time in the skillet when bacon fat is hot.

5. Cook for 4-5 minutes on each side.

6. Remove from the pan, let rest for 3-5 minutes.

7. Serve with extra cheese, bacon and onion if you want.

Nutrition per serving

- Calorie 433
- Carbs 1.2g
- Fat 34.5g
- Protein 29g

Bacon, Cauliflower and Cheddar Casserole

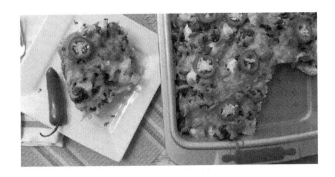

Ingredients for 6 servings

Ground Beef Mixture

- o   1/4 tsp. all-seasoning
- o   1/4 tsp. Onion Powder
- o   1 lb. Ground Beef (80/20)
- o   1 tsp. fish Sauce
- o   1 tbsp. Reduced Sugar Ketchup
- o   2 tsp. Minced Garlic
- o   1/2 tsp. Paprika
- o   1 tsp. Cumin
- o   1/2 tsp. Chili Powder
- o   1 tbsp. Soy Sauce

- 1/4 tsp. Cayenne Pepper

- 1 tbsp. Bacon Fat

- 1/4 tsp. Ground Black Pepper

- 1/2 tsp. Salt

Casserole Ingredients

- 1 medium Head Cauliflower, cut into florets

- 4 oz. Cheddar Cheese

- 10 oz. Bacon, chopped and fried

- 4 oz. Cream Cheese

Method

1. Except fish sauce, soy sauce and ketchup, thoroughly mix the ground beef with spices and seasoning. When mixed, put the mixture in a Ziploc bag and add the soy sauce, fish sauce, and ketchup.

2. Tightly roll the mixture inside the bag. Seal the bag and place in the fridge for minimum 30 minutes.

3. Chop bacon into pieces and pan fry them until crisp. Save the bacon grease

and place the bacon on paper towel to cool.

4. Add ground beef mixture to the pan and start to brown.

5. Now cut cauliflower into florets.

6. Preheat the oven to 350F. Arrange florets in the bottom of a casserole dish, then add ground beef and place chunks of cream cheese on top.

7. Now add the bacon, cheddar cheese, and pour the bacon grease on top.

8. Bake for 40-50 minutes, or until cheese is completely melted and browned on top.

Nutrition per serving

- o Calorie 575
- o Carbs 4.4g
- o Fat 46.3g
- o Protein 26.8g

Chapter 6 Dessert Recipes

Whip Cream and Coconut Milk Yogurt

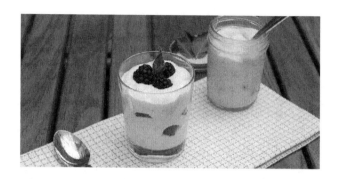

Ingredients for 2.3 cups (550ml) of yogurt

- ○ 1 can Full Fat Coconut Milk

- ○ 1/2 tsp. NOW Xanthan Gum

- ○ 2 capsules NOW Probiotic-10

- ○ 2/3 cup Heavy Whipping Cream

- ○ Toppings of Your Choice

Method

1. Stir a can of coconut milk, then pour the milk into two 200ml mason jars.

2. Add the contents of the probiotic capsules to the mason jars.

3. Place the mason jars in the oven for 12 to 24 hours, keep the oven light on and don't open the oven door. The mixture becomes thicker with time.

4. Once finished, pour the mixture into a mixing bowl.

5. Now ½ tsp. xanthan gum to the yogurt, then mix well with a hand blender. The mixture should be thick after this.

6. Whip heavy cream until stiff peaks form, in another bowl. Make it solid.

7. Add heavy cream to the yogurt and mix on low speed.

Nutrition per serving

- Calorie 315
- Carbs 4.3g
- Fat 31.3g
- Protein 0g

Organic Coconut Custard

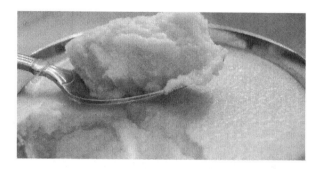

Ingredients for 4 large ramekins full of custard

- o 1/3 Cup Erythritol
- o 1 Cup Unsweetened Organic Coconut Milk
- o 1/3 Cup Macadamia Nut Butter
- o 4 Large Eggs
- o 1/3 Cup Heavy Cream
- o 1 tsp. Liquid Stevia
- o 1 tsp. Vanilla Extract

Method

1. Preheat the oven to 325F.

2. In a medium bowl, add coconut milk and heavy cream, now add vanilla extract.

3. Add 4 eggs, gently whisk together to avoiding aerating the eggs.

4. Add sweeteners and macadamia nut butter.

5. Stir continuously and make sure everything is combined and mixed evenly.

6. Fill a baking pan with 1-inch water.

7. Put the ramekins in the baking pan, ensure that water covers about 1 inch of the ramekins.

8. Fill the ramekins with the mixture.

9. Put the ramekins in the oven. Bake for 40 minutes or until a knife comes out clean.

10. When baked, remove from the oven, keep them in the water and allow to cool for 30 minutes.

11. Remove the ramekins from the water and serve.

Nutrition per serving

- ○ Calorie 275
- ○ Carbs 2.5g
- ○ Fat 26.2g
- ○ Protein 6.2g

Almond Chocolate and Peanut Butter Mug Cake

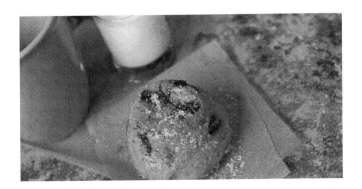

Ingredients for 1 mug cake

Base
- o   1 Tbsp. NOW Erythritol
- o   1 Large Egg
- o   2 Tbsp. Butter
- o   7 Drops Liquid Stevia
- o   2 Tbsp. Honeyville Almond Flour
- o   1/2 tsp. Baking Powder

Flavor

- o   1 Tbsp. Peanut Butter
- o   1/2 tsp. Vanilla Extract
- o   1 Bar (10g) Chocoperfection Dark Chocolate

Method

1. In a mug, mix together 2 tbsp. butter and 1 egg.
2. Add one 10g chunked Chocoperfection bar, 2 tbsp. almond flour, 1 tbsp. Now erythritol, ½ tsp. vanilla extract, ½ tsp. baking powder, 7 drops liquid stevia.
3. Mix the ingredients and add 1 tbsp. peanut butter, again mix everything.
4. Microwave on high for 65 seconds.
5. Remove the mug from the microwave. Place the mug upside down on a plate, bang it gently and the cake should smoothly come out of the mug.

Nutrition per serving

o   Calorie 488
o   Carbs 5g
o   Fat 47g
o   Protein 13g

Conclusion

Follow the ketogenic diet and live a healthy life.

35347064R00031

Made in the USA
San Bernardino, CA
21 June 2016